THE OBESITY CURE:

HOW TO CURB FOOD CRAVINGS, BURY POUND AND GAIN STRENGHT.

By

Edward S. Carson

Legal and disclaimer

The information containing in this book is not designed to replace or take the place of any form of medicine or professional medical advice. The information in this book has been provided for educational purpose only.

The information contain in this book has been compiled from sources deemed reliable, and it's accurate to the best of the authors knowledge; however the author cannot guarantee its accuracy and validity and cannot be held liable for any errors or omissions.

TABLE OF CONTENTS

INTRODUCTION

Obesity is outlined as Associate in nursing excessive accumulation of animal tissue compared to lean tissue. Technically, an individual is taken into account corpulent once his body mass index (BMI) is bigger than thirty. To know the importance of this downside from a health purpose of read, one simply ought to suppose that some years past, the WHO outlined fat mutually of the most important public health issues within the world along with temperature change. Solely within the u. s., common fraction of adults AR corpulent, whereas over a billion individuals worldwide AR overweight (and three hundred million of those AR obese).

Obesity ends up in a better risk to develop major chronic diseases like disorder, stroke, diabetes, some cancers (endometrial, colorectal, kidney, pancreas, breast, esophagus), Venice sickness, degenerative arthritis. Alternative issues related to this sickness AR depicted by high vital sign, high sterol, metabolic process issues, inflated surgical risk, gestation complications, hirsutism, discharge irregularities.

In several European countries the prevalence of fat has tripled since the 80s. The social value of this condition is currently adequate to 6 June 1944 of health care prices in

Europe. Fat is additionally the foremost common childhood disorder in Europe (20% of overweight youngsters of that one third obese).

Abdominal fat and vessel risk

Many studies show that abdominal fat is related to variety of negative consequences, among that Associate in Nursing inflated vessel risk, a better risk of developing polygenic disorder, that successively will increase the vessel risk, Associate in Nursing inflated cancer risk. The danger for the vascular system comes from the surplus fat within the abdomen that becomes dangerous once waist circumference exceeds eighty-eight cm in ladies or 102 cm in men. The abdominal animal tissue has a vigorous metabolic role. For instance, it produced:

substances that may promote the formation of plaques;

substances that favor endocrine resistance and promote the event of diabetes;

free fatty acids that act on the liver, increase endocrine resistance and alter the degree of fat and sugar within the blood;

substances that may trigger inflammatory processes that cause the formation and progression of plaque within the arteries.

Chapter 1

What Induced Obesity?

Obesity is one in every of the largest health issues within the world.

It's related to many connected conditions, put together referred to as metabolic syndrome. These embody high pressure, elevated glucose and a poor blood lipide profile. People with metabolic syndrome square measure at a far higher risk of cardiopathy and sort polygenic disease, compared to those whose weight is in a very normal range.

Over the past decades, a lot of analysis has centered on the causes of fleshiness and the way it may well be prevented or treated.

4 MAJOR CAUSES OF FLESHINESS

Genetics: Obesity encompasses a robust genetic part. Youngsters folks of oldsters of fogeys} with fleshiness square measure way more probably to possess fleshiness than youngsters of lean parents.

That doesn't mean that fleshiness is totally planned.

What you eat will have a significant impact on that genes Ar expressed and that don't seem to be.
Non-industrialized societies quickly develop fleshiness after they begin intake a typical Western diet. Their genes didn’t modification, however the surroundings and also the signals they sent to their genes did.
Put simply, genetic elements do have an effect on your status to gaining weight. Studies on identical twins demonstrate this alright.

Food Addiction:

Many sugar-sweetened, high-fat junk foods stimulate the reward centers in your brain.
In fact, these foods AR typically compared to unremarkable abused medicine like alcohol, cocaine, plant toxin and cannabis.
Junk foods will cause addiction in inclined people. These individuals lose management over their intake behavior, like individuals scuffling with drunkenness losing management over their drinking behavior.
Addiction may be a complicated issue that may be terribly tough to beat. Once you become smitten by one thing, you lose your freedom of alternative and also the organic chemistry in your brain starts career the shots for you

Insulin:

Insulin could be a vital secretion that regulates energy storage, among different things.

One of its functions is to inform fat cells to store fat and to carry on to the fat they already carry.

The Western diet promotes endocrine resistance in several overweight and people with blubber. This elevates endocrine levels everywhere the body, inflicting energy to urge hold on in fat cells rather than being obtainable to be used.

While insulin's role in blubber is arguable, many studies counsel that prime endocrine levels have a causative role within the development of blubber.

One of easyst|the most effective} ways in which to lower your endocrine is to chop back on simple or refined carbohydrates whereas increasing fiber intake.

Not sleeping enough:

Some analysis has urged that missing sleep will increase the chance of gaining weight and developing blubber. Researchers reviewed study proof for over twenty-eight thousand kids and fifteen thousand adults within the UK from 1977 to 2012. They finished that sleep deprivation considerably inflated the chance of blubber in both adults and kids. The changes affected kids as young as five years recent.

The team prompt that sleep deprivation might result in avoirdupois as a result of it will result in secretion changes that increase craving.

When an individual doesn't sleep enough, their body produces gherkin that could be a secretion that stimulates craving. At constant time, an absence of sleep conjointly leads to a lower production of leptin that could be a secretion that suppresses craving.

Chapter 2:

Structuring a Diet for a properly Weight Loss:

Dieting for fat loss may be troublesome and nearly appear to be an unending journey; however it definitely ought not to be if you find out how to make a pleasurable and property diet set up. Despite what several assume, weight loss isn't forever concerning intense restriction and rigidity, however rather finding ways in which to higher management food intake whereas adjusting meals to be additional acceptable for your goals. Even though many of us assume forceful modification is needed, doing therefore can build weight loss way more troublesome and positively not gratifying. Finding ways in which to mitigate this problem is of the utmost importance for a good diet. In this article, I'll bite on some key strategies I've used with thousands of purchasers over the years to make sure pregnant weight loss that's truly gratifying and property.

6 Steps to making a bespoken Diet set up for Weight Loss:

Achieving permanent and lasting weight loss needs a thoughtful uptake set up. Your body wants the proper balance of nutrition and calories for sustained energy through workouts and daily activities. Maintaining that balance is that the key to losing fat and keeping it off over time. A roaring diet set up for weight loss combines the vitamins and minerals your body must build muscle and maintain energy in one convenient and delicious menu. Follow these steps to style a diet set up for weight loss that's specifically structured to support your way, goals, and habits.

STEP ONE: AVOID CALORIE TALLY DIET PLANS:

Typical diet plans set a daily calorie goal. Dieters are expected to stay their consumption at intervals a definite varies daily with meals that contain all the important nutrients their bodies ought to thrive. However, this foundational belief sets several dieters up for failure before they even begin. We tend to suggest an immensely totally different approach to calorie tally. Why could be a daily count the incorrect thanks to approach nutritional intake? Every food has totally different calorie content. Unless you eat nearly an equivalent issue daily, it gets troublesome to stay track of what proportion you're overwhelming while not arduous following. From payment day trip with friends to happening vacation, there are variety of times once dieters merely can't maintain a strict daily count while not sacrificing enjoyment of social things. To short-circuit temptation, several diet plans necessitate a "cheat day" that enables the dieter to eat no matter they need while not tally the calories. It's doable to stay to a daily restrictive calorie count and still not slim down because of overindulging sooner or later every week. Daily calorie counts tend to encourage under eating. Dieters try and keep underneath their limits to preserve caloric deficits. Over time, to several incomprehensible calories negatively impact weight loss efforts. Instead of setting yourself to a group variety of calories per day, we tend to suggest you develop a diet set up that covers your nutritional wants to take care of a healthy way. This approach is exceptionally useful during a weight loss program because it helps along with your energy levels, is a smaller amount restrictive, and permits you the liberty to fancy what you would like however sparsely. Decisive your organic process desires is completely different for each person supported their age, weight, activity levels, and alternative medical desires. Setting these organic process goals or pointers provides you the pliability to eat a range of various foods to succeed in your weight loss goals. These organic process goals specialize in your intake levels of: super molecule, carbs, fats, vitamins, and minerals. Keeping these key factors balanced for what your body desires may be an additional no-hit approach for weight loss than calories numeration.

STEP TWO: CALCULATE YOUR MACROS:

Dieting isn't on the subject of what quantity you eat. You furthermore might have to be compelled to make sure that you're giving your body what it has to grow muscle, melt fat, and keep your energy high. Macronutrients area unit the essential building blocks your body uses to accomplish these tasks. These basic nutrients additionally represent the majority of your caloric intake.

The 3 main classes for macros are:

Carbohydrates: Easy and sophisticated sugar chains break down within the body to supply fuel for muscles.

Fats: Excess calories area unit hold on in fat cells to supply emergency energy once fast-burning carbs aren't obtainable.

Fat it is a necessary part in several secretion and brain functions similarly.

Proteins: These powerhouse macros give property energy and material want to repair and grow tissues throughout the body. Balancing these macronutrients provides you the most effective likelihood of building the body you would like while not feeling disadvantaged or exhausted. The overall rule of thumb suggests that you just divide your calorie intake into thirty-fifth healthy fat, four-hundredth super molecule, and twenty-fifth carbohydrates. For an additional personalized quantitative relation, use an internet calculator to see your best combine.

STEP THREE: REALIZE FOODS THAT MATCH:

Once you recognize what quantity you wish to eat, pay your time finding foods that match into your new fashion. An efficient diet arranges for weight loss should embrace foods that you'll really eat. If you don't fancy what you're ingestion, it's unlikely that you'll continue your arrangement. However, it's additionally vital to place some effort into attempting new menu choices. Several dieters come back to weight loss programs as a result of a restricted diet that's high in empty calories. Adding additional organic process choices to your daily menu is a necessary step to making a long-run ingestion arrange. Start by creating an inventory of the foods and ingredients that you just love the foremost. Once your diet begins, aim to feature one or two new fruits, vegetables, or grain alternatives hebdomadally to your list. It's useful to additionally embrace knowledge on the macronutrient content of every item, as this can assist you decide what quantity every of every} of those ingredients you'll fancy in each meal.

STEP FOUR: REPLENISH ON RECIPES: Now that you just recognize what you'll eat, begin aggregation a range of recipes that feature your listed foods. Concentrate to preparation directions. The approach you cook your food features a massive impact on macronutrient content. A large instruction choice is vital in your diet arrange for weight loss as a result of it keeps you from losing interest. Losing interest in daily menus is that the main reason several dieters don't reach their goals. Selection ensures that you'll forever forestall to your next serving. An internet instruction book may be a good way to store your recipes. With enough analysis, you'll tailor your instruction assortment to suit your preferences. Area unit you a devotee of sweetbreads and pastries? Realize low-calorie versions of your favorite food. Area unit sauces a necessary a part of your daily feeding experience? Rummage around for home-baked versions of your most often used condiments. Will the thought of discarding deep-fried foods cause you to nervous? Rummage around for recipes that use your kitchen appliance to simulate the crunchiness you crave while not the extra fat content. For people who live life on-the-go, compile an inventory of your most frequented restaurants. Raise the workers for organic process info on their menu things. Use that knowledge to make an inventory of alternatives that match at intervals your dietary budget.

STEP FIVE: SET AN INGESTION SCHEDULE:

When you eat is simply as vital as what you eat. Our bodies undergo cycles day after day that have an effect on our ability to metabolize abdomen contents. Also, existing medical conditions or variations in body functions will modification the approach you method meals. For many, a diet arrange for weight loss that follows the standard three meals daily paradigm doesn't work. This can be very true for people who area unit sharply reducing their daily calorie intake. Strive spacing your meals and snacks roughly three hours apart. This keeps you from obtaining too hungry and running for unhealthy choices to fill your belly. Here area unit another pointers to assist you build the proper diet arrange for weight loss. Eat a filling dinner to avoid late night snacking. Consume a high-protein breakfast at intervals AN hour of wakening. Stick to your regular plan. If you have got polygenic disease or alternative aldohexose conditions that area unit wedged by your ingestion habits, see your doctor for facilitate building a schedule that helps maintain the right glucose levels.

STEP SIX: TRACK, ANALYZE, AND ADJUST:

Use a food diary to stay track of your plan. This creates a record that enables you to go back your ingestion habits and analyze the effectiveness of your arrangement. Build changes once required to stay you not off course to your goal weight. Don't be afraid to alter things up if a particular dietary arrange isn't providing the specified results.

CHAPTER 3

The secretion structures of fat:

Hormones that have an effect on Your Weight — and the way to enhance them Hormones square measure vital substances that function chemical messengers in your body. They facilitate nearly each activity, together with metabolism, hunger, and fullness. As a result of their association with craving, some hormones additionally play a big role in weight.

HERE SQUARE MEASURE FIVE HORMONES WHICH WILL HAVE AN EFFECT ON YOUR WEIGHT, AND THE SIDE TIPS FOR KEEPING THEM AT HEALTHY LEVELS

1. **Insulin:** Insulin, the most storage secretion in your body, is made by your duct gland. In healthy people, internal secretion promotes the storage of aldohexose — an easy sugar you get from food — within the muscle, liver, and fat cells for later use. Your body secretes internal secretion in tiny amounts throughout the day and in larger amounts when meals. This secretion then transfers aldohexose from food into your cells for either

energy or storage, betting on your body's current wants. Insulin resistance could be a fairly common condition that causes your cells to prevent responding to internal secretion. This condition leads too high {blood sugar|blood aldohexose|glucose} as a result of the internal secretion cannot move glucose into your cells. Your duct gland then produces even a lot of internal secretion in a shot to spice up aldohexose absorption. Insulin resistance has been coupled to fat, that successively will play a task in alternative conditions, like kind two polygenic disorder and heart condition. Insulin sensitivity is thought of because the opposite of internal secretion resistance. It means that your cells square measure sensitive to internal secretion. Thus, it's an honest plan to concentrate on life-style habits that facilitate improve internal secretion sensitivity, like the subsequent. Tips to enhance internal secretion sensitivity Exercise frequently. Analysis supports exercise, at each high and moderate intensities, as a method of up internal secretion sensitivity and decreasing internal secretion resistance. Improve your sleep habits. Not obtaining enough sleep, or not obtaining quality sleep, is coupled to fat and internal secretion resistance. Get a lot of polyunsaturated fatty acid fatty acids. Analysis indicates that polyunsaturated fatty acid supplements could improve internal secretion sensitivity in folks with metabolic conditions like polygenic disorder. If you aren't a devotee of supplements, strive consumption a lot of fish, nuts, seeds, and plant oils. Change your diet. The Mediterranean diet — which has several veggies, yet as healthy fats from loony and extra-virgin vegetable oil — could facilitate cut back internal secretion resistance. Decreasing your intake of saturated and trans fats might also facilitate. Maintain a moderate weight. In folks with overweight, healthy weight loss and weight management could improve internal secretion sensitivity. Focus on low glycemic carbs. Instead of try and eliminate carbs from your diet, aim to create most of them low glycemic and high fiber. Examples embrace whole grains, fruits, vegetables, and legumes.

2. Leptin:

Leptin could be a fullness secretion that works by telling your neural structure — the portion of your brain that regulates craving — that you're full. However, folks with fat could expertise leptin resistance. This implies the message to prevent consumption doesn't reach your brain, eventually inflicting you to gormandize. In turn, your body could turn out even a lot of leptin till your levels become elevated. The direct reason behind leptin resistance is unclear, however it should result to inflammation, citron mutations, and/or excessive leptin production, which might occur with fat. Tips to enhance leptin levels Although no renowned treatment exists for leptin resistance, some life-style changes could facilitate lower leptin levels. Maintain a healthy weight. As a result of leptin resistance is related to fat, it's vital to keep up a healthy weight. To boot, analysis suggests that a decrease in body fat could facilitate cut back leptin levels. Improve your sleep quality. Leptin levels are also associated with sleep quality in individuals with fat. Though this association might not exist in individuals while not fat, there AR various different reasons to urge higher sleep. Exercise frequently. Analysis links regular, consistent exercise to a decrease in leptin levels.

3. Ghrelin:

Ghrelin is basically the other of leptin. It's the hunger endocrine that sends a message to your neural structure indicating that your abdomen is empty and wishes food. Its main perform is to extend pretence. Normally, internal secretion levels ar highest before uptake and lowest when a meal. Curiously, analysis indicates that individuals with fat have low internal secretion levels however AR a lot of sensitive to its effects. This sensitivity might result in deadly sin. Tips to manage internal secretion levels One reason weight loss typically will be|is|may be} tough is that limiting calories often results in accrued internal secretion levels, going you hungry. In addition, metabolism tends to weigh down and leptin levels decrease. As such, here Ar some tips for lowering internal secretion to assist cut back appetite: Maintain a moderate weight. Fat might increase your sensitivity to internal secretion, ultimately increasing your pretence. Try to get sensible quality sleep. Poor sleep might result in will increase in internal secretion, overeating, and weight gain. Eat frequently. As a result of internal secretion levels ar highest before a meal, hear your body and eat once you're hungry. People with fat might become a lot of sensitive to the results of the hunger endocrine internal secretion. Analysis suggests that maintaining a moderate weight and prioritizing sleep facilitate with managing this endocrine.

4. Cortisol: Cortisol is thought because the stress endocrine and is created by your adrenal glands. During times of stress, this endocrine triggers a rise in rate and energy levels. The discharge of corticosteroid — aboard the endocrine endocrine — is often referred to as the "fight or flight" response. While it's necessary for yours to body unharnessed corticosteroid in dangerous things, chronic high levels might result in several health problems, as well as cardiomyopathy, diabetes, low energy levels, high vital sign, sleep disturbances, and weight gain. Certain modus vivendi factors — as well as poor sleep habits, chronic stress, and a high intake of high glycemic foods — might contribute to high corticosteroid levels. Plus, not solely will fat raise corticosteroid levels, however high levels may additionally cause weight gain, making a feedback loop.

Tips for lowering corticosteroid levels Here are some modus vivendi changes that will facilitate manage corticosteroid levels:

Optimize sleep: Chronic sleep problems, as well as sleep disorder, sleep disorder, and irregular sleep habits (like those of shift workers), might contribute to high corticosteroid levels. Target developing a daily hour and sleep schedule.

Exercise frequently. Corticosteroid levels briefly increase when high intensity exercise, however regular exercise typically helps decrease levels by rising overall health and lowering stress levels. Practice attentiveness. analysis suggests that frequently active attentiveness lowers corticosteroid levels, though' a lot of analysis is

required. Attempt adding meditation to your daily routine.
Maintain a moderate weight. As a result of fat might increase corticosteroid levels and high corticosteroid levels will cause weight gain, maintaining a moderate weight might facilitate keep levels in restraint.
Eat a diet. Analysis has shown that diets high in supplemental sugars, refined grains, and saturated fat might result in higher corticosteroid levels. in addition, following the Mediterranean diet might facilitate lower corticosteroid levels.

5. Estrogen: Estrogen may be an endocrine to blame for regulation the feminine genital system, still because the immune, skeletal, and tube systems.
Levels of this endocrine modification throughout life stages like gestation, nursing, and change of life, still as throughout the oscillation. High levels of estrogen, that Ar typically seen in individuals with fat, ar related to associate in nursing accrued risk of sure cancers and different chronic diseases. Conversely, low levels — usually seen with aging, perimenopause, and change of life — might have an effect on weight and body fat, so additionally increasing your risk of chronic ailments. Individuals with low estrogen levels typically expertise

central fat, that is Associate in nursing accumulation of weight round the trunk of the body. this will cause alternative health issues, like high blood glucose, high vital sign, and heart condition. You can lower your risk of the many of those health conditions through manner changes — particularly by maintaining a healthy weight. **Tips to keep up healthy steroid hormone levels:** To keep steroid hormone levels at a healthy equilibrium, strive a number of these techniques: Try to manage your weight. Weight loss or maintenance might scale back the chance of heart condition because of low steroid hormone levels in girls ages 55–75. analysis conjointly supports healthy weight maintenance for reducing your tie of chronic diseases generally.

CHAPTER 4

HOW TO LOSE FAT NOT MUSCLE:

How to Lose Fat while not Losing Muscle Losing fat Maintaining muscle Exercise, plans Healthy uptake, Talk with a professional Takeaway If you've been operating laborious to induce in form nonetheless still need to lose fat, you'll have considerations that you'll lose muscle furthermore. To forestall this, you'll be able to follow a number of uptake and fitness pointers that may assist you bring home the bacon the results you would like. You must approach losing weight safely and effectively to optimize fat loss and muscle maintenance. This is often particularly necessary if you would like to keep up your fitness level, physical activity, and overall perform. With the correct approach, it's potential to lose fat whereas maintaining muscle mass. This text outlines however you'll be able to use associate degree exercise and uptake conceive to effectively shed fat while not losing muscle.

What it takes to lose fat: To lose fat, you would like to consume fewer calories than you burn on a daily basis and exercise frequently. Frequent physical activities helps get eliminate fat. If you reduce while not exercise, you're additional doubtless to lose each muscle and fat. While it’s insufferable to lose fat on specific areas of your body, you'll be able to work on lowering your overall body fat proportion. Go slowly. Losing weight quickly could contribute to muscle loss. It’s best to lose a tiny low quantity of weight hebdomadally over an extended amount.

How to maintain muscle: To keep the muscle you have got whereas losing fat, you’ll get to strike a balance between limiting yourself and pushing yourself the maximum amount as you'll be able to. Each person can have completely different results. Hear your body, and change your exercising and uptake arrange consequently. **Schedule recovery time:** Give yourself enough time to recover between workouts. This is often particularly necessary if your uptake fewer calories and doing intense workouts. Get much sleep that helps restore your energy levels.

Don’t limit. Avoid any form of uptake arrange that’s too forceful or restrictive. It'll be more durable to stay up with future. Avoid overtraining, and keep one's distance from any exercising arrange that has the potential to empty you or cause injury. Pushing yourself too laborious or quick could end in missing workouts because of fatigue or injury. Remember, rest days square measure necessary.

Exercise: Exercise is another necessary side of maintaining muscle mass, with resistance, endurance, or each variety of coaching in older adults with avoirdupois. The researchers found that once people followed associate degree uptake arrange and did some form of exercise, they were ready to forestall muscle loss because of calorie restriction. Most of the uptake plans consisted of fifty-five % carbohydrates, fifteen % macromolecule, and thirty % fat. More analysis is required to work out which kind of exercise is only in preventing muscle loss.

Eat healthy: Change up your uptake conceive to embody healthy proteins and fewer unhealthy fat sources. Researchers found older adults maintained additional lean mass and lost additional fat once intense higher macromolecule diets.

Try a supplement: Consider taking a supplement, like atomic number 24 picoliter that is claimed to own a positive result on weight loss, hunger, and blood glucose levels. Eating the correct amounts of macronutrients, like proteins, fats, and carbohydrates managing calorie intake Doing resistance exercise before taking any supplement, it's an honest plan to ascertain in together with your doctor. Some supplements could negatively move with sure medications or conditions. Exercise plans follow a number of those tips to assist you exercise smarter to hit your goals.

Do cardio: To lose fat and gain or maintain muscle mass, do moderate- to high-intensity cardio for a minimum of a hundred and fifty minutes per week. Example of cardio exercises include: Cycling, Running, Boxing, Soccer Basketball, Volleyball.

Increase intensity: Increase the intensity of your workouts to challenge yourself and burn calories. For your exercising to effectively build strength, you want to push your muscles to their most capability. This might involve taking an opportunity before continuing.
Continue to strength train: Do strength coaching to a few times per week. This might be a mix of: Weightlifting Body weight exercises, Resistance band exercises. Exercise categories, like yoga, Pilates, or tai chi, are choices. Always begin with low weight masses and fewer repetitions. Step by step work yourself far to heavier weights or additional repetitions. This can facilitate avoid injury. Strength coaching helps forestall muscle loss

whereas increasing muscle mass. Certify your routine is balanced and targets all the most muscle teams. Give your muscle teams time to recover. You'll be able to aim to focus on every muscle group A most double per week. To cut fat, you'll be able to additionally incorporate interval coaching into your exercising arrange. Take a rest Allow for adequate rest and recovery on alternate days. Either take a whole day without work, or elect light-intensity exercise, like walking, swimming, or dancing. 6. Neuropeptide Y Neuropeptide Y (NPY) may be an internal secretion created by cells in your brain and system that stimulates appetence and reduces energy expenditure in response to abstinence or stress. Because it's going to stimulate food intake, NPY is related to blubber and weight gain. It's activated in fat tissue and should increase fat storage and cause abdominal blubber and metabolic syndrome, a condition that may increase the chance of chronic diseases. Research has shown that NPY's mechanisms that cause blubber might also cause associate inflammatory response, any worsening health condition.

Tips for maintaining low NPY levels Here square measure some tips for maintaining healthy levels of NPY:

Exercise: Some studies counsel that regular exercise might facilitate decrease NPY levels, tho' analysis is mixed.

Eat a nourishing diet. Though a lot of analysis is required, high fat, high sugar diets might increase NPY levels — thus you'll wish to contemplate lowering your intake of foods high in sugar and fat. 7. Glucagon-like peptide-1 Glucagon-like peptide-1 (GLP-1) may be an internal secretion created in your gut once nutrients enter your intestines. It plays a significant role keep blood glucose levels stable and creating you're feeling full. Research suggests that individuals with blubber might have issues with GLP-1 sign. As such, GLP-1 is accessories to medications — notably for individuals with polygenic disorder — to cut back weight and waist circumference.

Tips for keeping GLP-1 levels under control Here square measure some tips to assist maintain healthy levels of GLP-1: **Eat much macromolecule**. High macromolecule foods like whey macromolecule and dairy product are shown to extend GLP-1 levels. Consider taking probiotics. Preliminary analysis suggests that probiotics might increase GLP-1 levels, though' a lot of human analysis is required. To boot, it's best to talk with a care skilled before beginning any new supplements. 8. Cholecystokinin Like GLP-1, cholecystokinin (CCK) may be a fullness internal secretion created by cells in your gut when a meal. It's vital for energy production, macromolecule synthesis, digestion, and alternative bodily functions. It conjointly will increase the discharge of the fullness internal secretion leptin. People with blubber might have a reduced sensitivity to CCK's effects, which can cause chronic gula. In turn, this could any scale back CCK sensitivity, making a feedback loop. **Tips for increasing CCK levels, Here square measure some tips for maintaining healthy levels of CCK:**

1. **Eat much macromolecule**. Some analysis suggests a high macromolecule diet might facilitate increase CCK levels, and thus fullness.
2. **Exercise**. Whereas analysis is proscribed, some proof supports regular exercise for increasing CCK levels. Peptide YY Peptide YY (PYY) is another gut internal secretion that decreases appetence. PYY levels could also be lower in individuals with

blubber, and this could cause a bigger appetence and gala. Decent levels square measure believed to play a significant role in reducing food intake and decreasing the chance of blubber. **Tips for raising PYY levels Here square measure some ways that to stay PYY at a healthy level in your body**: Follow an all-round diet. Consumption much macromolecule might promote healthy PYY levels and fullness. To boot, the paleo diet — which incorporates ample macromolecule, fruits, and veggies — might raise PYY levels, however a lot of analysis is required.

CONCLUSION

The blubber Code may be a timely browse that gives insight into what has slowly evolved into a scourge in today's society-blubber. It delves into the present myths on weight loss and offers unbelievable insights into factors that result in blubber.

A review of key takeaways includes:

1. A calorie deficit isn't a primary driver for weight loss.
2. Carbohydrate, and significantly sugar, is accountable for excessive weight gain.

3. The food business is part accountable for the rise in blubber.

4. Hormones, specifically hormone, square measure accountable for weight gain and integral to weight loss.

5. Low-carb, mid-protein diets square measure best if weight loss is that the goal.

6. Intermittent abstinence is crucial keep hormone at the optimum levels.

7. Substitute adscititious sugars, processed foods, and easy carbs with healthy fats, fibers, and vinegar.

www.ingramcontent.com/pod-product-compliance
Lightning Source LLC
LaVergne TN
LVHW020537160826
845677LV00015B/4115
* 9 7 9 8 3 6 6 4 8 6 6 3 7 *